I0846153

SCIATICA RELIEF FOR SENIORS

AMANDA WATSON

COPYRIGHT © 2026 BY AMANDA WATSON

ISBN-13 979-8856979298

All rights reserved.

No portion of this book may be reproduced in any form without written permission from the publisher or author, except as permitted by U.S. copyright law.

This publication is designed to provide accurate and authoritative information in regard to the subject matter covered. It is sold with the understanding that neither the author nor the publisher is engaged in rendering legal, investment, accounting or other professional services.

While the publisher and author have used their best efforts in preparing this book, they make no representations or warranties with respect to the accuracy or completeness of the contents of this book and specifically disclaim any implied warranties of merchantability or fitness for a particular purpose.

No warranty may be created or extended by sales representatives or written sales materials. The advice and strategies contained herein may not be suitable for your situation. You should consult with a professional when appropriate.

Neither the publisher nor the author shall be liable for any loss of profit or any other commercial damages, including but not limited to special, incidental, consequential, personal, or other damages.

Disclaimer

The information provided in this book is intended to be educational and supportive.

It is not a substitute for professional medical advice, diagnosis, or treatment.

The author and publisher are not medical professionals; the content is based on research, personal experience, and general field knowledge.

Before attempting any of the natural treatments or strategies outlined in this book, it is strongly recommended that you consult with a qualified healthcare professional, such as a physician, physical therapist, or other medical practitioner.

Each individual health condition is unique, and what may work for one person may not be suitable for another,

The author and publisher do not assume any responsibility for any harm, injury, or adverse effect resulting from using the information presented in this book. The contents is intended as a general guide and starting point for those seeking natural approaches to managing sciatic pain, particularly seniors. It is essential to use caution, listen to your body, and seek medical guidance when necessary.

Any reliance on the information provided in this book is at your discretion and risk.

By reading this book, you acknowledge and agree to the terms of this disclaimer. If you have any concerns about your health or the treatments or suitability, please consult a healthcare professional before changing your health regime.

Contents

1. Introduction — 1

2. A Brief Explanation of Age-Related Sciatic Factors — 7

3. A Triad for Relief in Seniors — 11

4. Nurturing Flexibility and Mobility for Seniors — 15

5. A Holistic Approach to Pain Management — 25

6. Herbal and Supplement Remedies — 31

7. Nature's Soothing Tonic for Relief — 35

8. Acupuncture, Acupressure, Chiropractic Remedies — 39

9. Yoga, Tai Chi, and the Art of Integration — 43

10. A Guide to Ergonomic Aids — 53

11. Conclusion — 59

Resource — 63

Books in this Series — 67

CHAPTER 1

INTRODUCTION

As we age, our bodies undergo various changes that can impact our overall well-being, and one common issue that many seniors face is sciatica. You may feel it will only worsen as you age and cannot be reversed.

After all, 80 percent of all American adults suffer from some form or other of back pain.

Well, I am here to tell you that is a depressing thought, and this crippling pain can be managed and even disappear.

Sciatica affects both men and women and is characterized by pain radiating along the sciatic nerve. It can be debilitating and significantly affect daily life.

In this book, we will investigate some of the options to reduce this debilitating pain that significantly affects everyday life.

While conventional medical treatments indeed have their place, there's a growing awareness of the importance of addressing sciatica naturally, especially for seniors, so we will also explore why natural remedies matter and how they can positively impact seniors' well-being.

Healing Starts With You
Buried within you, like everyone else on this planet, you have the energy and power to heal yourself. However, it has to be said that not everyone heals at the same rate. For example, a small paper cut may take longer to heal in some people than in others. Sometimes, even people no longer realize they still have this power to reduce pain. Throughout this journey, you must always stay optimistic and remember that you have the power to heal yourself. In doing so, your body will improve at healing, and you will begin to enjoy an active and pain-free lifestyle regardless of age. However, you must seek a medical professional's guidance if you hurt yourself.

Misconception of Your Pain

- Pain is our enemy – Pain is natural, and your brain warns you that something is wrong with your body.

- Pain will only ever go when you take Painkillers. Remember that pain's prime purpose is to mask a problem. Indeed, with some such medications, the side effects can be shocking, leading to liver damage, increased blood heart, and strain on the heart.

- The Surgeon's Knife is the Only Answer - This is untrue, should be the last resort, and carries its own risks. It is not a quick fix!

- You Should Rest as You are Pain - Pain should not hold you back from reasonable activities. In many cases, such action will lead to increased joint problems. Restricting such moves will only deprive your body of the necessary physical activity. That said, taking time to let a muscle recover after trauma is advisable under the guidance of your doctor. Still, it will deprive the muscle of the regular activity it needs to repair itself.

- Lifting causes Sciatica and Lower Back Problems. Lifting incorrectly is undoubtedly a route to back problems in the future. If an item is too heavy, use a suitable mechanical device or the help of a colleague. Always remember to keep the back straight and lift with your knees, not your back or arms.

- My Back Pain is the result of an injury – By the time our backs develop pain, we will most likely have endured several tens of years of wear. The human spine can absorb an exceptional amount of energy without damage. Back pain may result from a recent injury, usually healing within six months. If this is not the case, then consult a medical professional.

- There is a perfect cure for my chronic back pain – We are all different, so the conception of "a perfect cure with straightforward medication" is not valid! We can not turn off our pain receptors without damaging other vital functions, for, as we said earlier, they are the brain's way of signalling that something is wrong. The correct and only way forward is to address the root cause of your pain by focusing on joint flexibility and muscle health through exercise.

Holistic Approach to Health

Natural treatments emphasize a holistic approach to health, which is particularly relevant for seniors. Instead of merely alleviating symptoms, natural remedies aim to address the underlying causes of sciatica. Seniors often have multiple health concerns, and addressing sciatica can contribute to their overall well-being by promoting a healthier lifestyle that considers factors such as diet, exercise, and mental health.

Risk of Side Effects

Conventional medical treatments, including medications and visits to surgeries, can sometimes come with unwanted side effects, which may be more pronounced in older adults.

On the other hand, natural therapies often involve fewer risks of adverse reactions. Seniors are typically more sensitive to medications and medical interventions, making natural alternatives a safer option for managing sciatica without the potential complications of pharmaceuticals.

- Preservation of Mobility and Independence Seniors cherish their independence, and sciatica can hinder mobility. Natural treatments focusing on gentle exercises, stretches, and lifestyle adjustments can help maintain or improve mobility. By addressing sciatica naturally, seniors can continue to engage in activities they enjoy, maintain their social connections, and avoid the loss of independence that often accompanies chronic pain.

- Comprehensive Pain Management - Sciatica can cause physical discomfort and emotional distress. Natural treatments encompass pain management techniques, including relaxation exercises, mindfulness, and meditation. These techniques not only alleviate physical pain but also contribute to emotional well-being. For seniors who may already be dealing with emotional challenges, a holistic approach that targets both the body and mind can have profound positive effects.

- Empowerment Through Self-Care Seniors who actively participate in their health management often feel more empowered and in control of their well-being. Natural treatments require seniors to take an active role in their healing journey. This empowerment can boost self-esteem and confidence, fostering a sense of accomplishment as they witness their efforts, resulting in pain relief and improved quality of life.

- Dependency on Medications - Many seniors already take multiple medications for various health conditions. Addressing sciatica can help reduce the need for additional medications to manage pain and, at the same time, can minimize potential drug interactions and adverse effects associated with pharmacy, leading to a more straightforward, more manageable health regime.

In conclusion, addressing sciatica can offer a holistic, personalized, and gentle approach to pain management for seniors. By focusing on natural treatments, seniors can experience relief from sciatic pain without the potential risks and side effects associated with conventional medical interventions.

More than just pain relief, natural approaches promote overall well-being, empower seniors to take charge of their health, and contribute to a higher quality of life as they continue to enjoy their golden years to the fullest.

CHAPTER 2

A BRIEF EXPLANATION OF AGE-RELATED SCIATIC FACTORS

Sciatica is a condition that affects people of all ages and becomes increasingly common and potentially more challenging in later life due to age-related factors. It can be highly uncomfortable and seriously impact your ability to do even simple tasks.

Understanding what sciatica is and how aging influences its development is essential to address this discomfort in older adults effectively.

So, *what is Sciatica?*

Sciatica is a word that doctors will use to describe several different symptoms in the leg. These symptoms can range from pain, numbness, weakness, or a tingling sensation. It can have other causes and flares up when the sciatic nerve is irritated in some way, most commonly by a herniated disc, bulging disc, or degenerative disk disease.

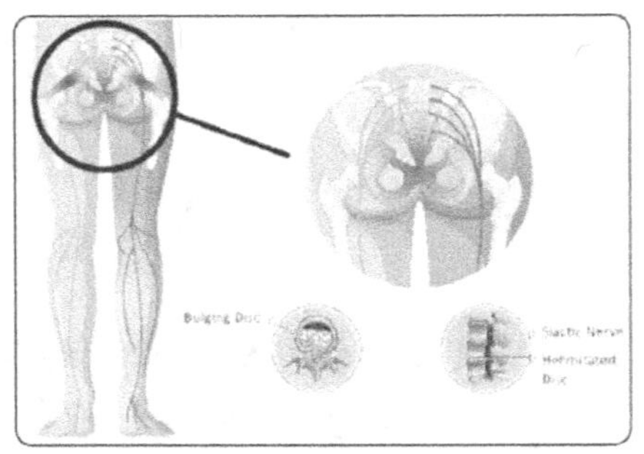

THE SCIATIC NERVE RUNS FROM THE LOWER SPINE
THROUGH THE BUTTOCKS AND DOWN BOTH LEGS.

Because it is so long, if you are experiencing sciatica, you may experience pain and symptoms throughout the entire nerve length. The pain can range from a mild ache to severe, sharp sensations, often accompanied by numbness, tingling, or weakness in the affected leg.

Sciatica is not a diagnosis but a symptom of an underlying issue, most commonly compression or irritation of the sciatic nerve. This sciatic pain in seniors can be caused by (but is not limited to) to:

- Degenerative Changes in the Spine - The spine undergoes natural wear and tear as we age. Our intervertebral discs, which act as cushions between the spinal vertebrae, tend to lose water content and become less flexible over time, leading to herniated discs and spinal stenosis.

- Herniated discs can protrude and press on the sciatic nerve, causing pain. Spinal stenosis, characterized by the narrowing of the spinal canal, can result in compression of the nerve roots that form the sciatic nerve.

- Changes in Bone Density - Seniors often experience decreased bone density, making them more susceptible to osteoporosis. Weakening bones can contribute to vertebral fractures or collapse, which can impinge on nerve roots and the sciatic nerve. Fractures can cause sudden onset sciatica or exacerbate pre-existing discomfort.

- Muscle Atrophy and Weakness - Aging can lead to muscle atrophy and weakness, mainly if seniors are less active. Weak muscles may fail to support the spine adequately, leading to poor posture and increased pressure on spinal structures. Poor posture can exacerbate sciatic pain by contributing to nerve compression or irritation.

- Reduced Elasticity of Soft Tissues – Connective tissues, such as ligaments and tendons, become less elastic as we age. This reduced elasticity can contribute to conditions like piriformis syndrome, where the piriformis muscle in the buttocks irritates the sciatic nerve. The likelihood of soft tissues causing sciatic pain increases as their flexibility diminishes.

- Inflammation and Circulation Issues Aging bodies often experience increased inflammation and reduced circulation. Inflammation can irritate nerves and exacerbate pain. Additionally, diminished circulation may hinder the delivery of nutrients and oxygen to nerve tissues, affecting their function and potentially causing pain along the sciatic nerve pathway.

- Accumulated Strain and Injuries - The spine can get strained throughout a lifetime from various activities, injuries, and poor postural habits. Over time, this strain can contribute to spinal issues like herniated discs or muscle imbalances that trigger sciatic pain, particularly in seniors with a history of physically demanding work or injuries.

- Other Health Conditions - Seniors are likelier to have pre-existing health conditions like diabetes or cardiovascular issues. These conditions can contribute to nerve damage or circulatory problems, increasing the risk of sciatic pain. Moreover, diseases like diabetes can impair nerve function, making the nerves more susceptible to compression.

Recognizing these age-related factors is crucial for effectively managing sciatic pain in older adults. By addressing these factors through natural treatments, exercise, and lifestyle adjustments, seniors can mitigate the impact of these changes and experience relief from sciatica for a better quality of life in their golden years.

In summary, in this chapter, we have discussed how sciatic pain in seniors is influenced by age-related changes in the spine, bones, muscles, and other bodily structures. The degenerative processes that occur as we age can contribute to conditions that impinge on or irritate the sciatic nerve, leading to discomfort.

Chapter 3

A Triad for Relief in Seniors

Sciatica, as we have discussed, is a condition that causes pain along the sciatic nerve and can be incredibly challenging for seniors. However, practical strategies can help manage and alleviate sciatic pain.

These strategies include maintaining a healthy weight, regular low-impact exercises, and improving posture and body mechanics. These three pillars work together synergistically to ease sciatic pain and enhance the overall well-being of seniors.

Maintaining a Healthy Weight
Carrying excess weight places additional stress on the spine and can exacerbate sciatic pain. In seniors, maintaining a healthy weight is not just about appearance; it directly impacts their spinal health and overall quality of life. Excess weight can contribute to herniated discs and spinal stenosis, which can compress the sciatic nerve. By shedding extra pounds, seniors can reduce the pressure on their spine and provide much-needed relief to the affected nerve.

Healthy weight management involves a balanced diet focusing on nutrient-dense foods, appropriate portions, and mindful eating habits. Seniors should incorporate plenty of fruits, vegetables, lean proteins, whole grains, and healthy fats.

It's essential to consult a healthcare professional or a registered dietitian to create a personalized eating plan that aligns with any underlying health conditions.

Incorporating Regular Low-Impact Exercises
Exercise is crucial in managing sciatica, but seniors must approach it carefully. Low-impact exercises are gentle on the joints and spine, making them suitable for seniors looking to alleviate sciatic pain. These exercises can help improve circulation, strengthen muscles, promote flexibility, improve spine health, and reduce sciatic discomfort.

Walking is one of the simplest and most effective low-impact exercises for seniors. It improves cardiovascular health, enhances circulation, and supports weight management. Swimming and water aerobics are also excellent options, as the buoyancy of water reduces the impact on joints while providing resistance for muscle strengthening.

Yoga and Tai Chi are gentle practices that combine movement, breath, and mindfulness. They help improve balance, flexibility, and posture—crucial to managing sciatica.

Before beginning any exercise regimen, seniors should consult their healthcare provider to ensure the chosen activities are safe and appropriate for their health.

Improving Posture and Body Mechanic
Proper posture and body mechanics are foundational to spine health and can significantly impact sciatic pain.

Seniors are more susceptible to poor posture due to age-related muscle and bone changes. Slouching or hunching forward stresses the spine and can compress the sciatic nerve, exacerbating pain. Seniors should maintain a neutral spine alignment during all activities, whether sitting, standing, or walking.

A chair with proper lumbar support can help keep a natural curve in the lower back. Distributing body weight evenly between both feet and engaging core muscles can alleviate pressure on the spine when standing.

Additionally, seniors should be mindful of their body mechanics during daily activities. Lifting objects with the legs rather than the back and avoiding twisting motions can prevent strains and reduce the risk of further aggravating sciatic pain.

The beauty of these three strategies—maintaining a healthy weight, incorporating regular low-impact exercises, and improving posture—is that they complement each other and create a holistic approach to managing sciatic pain in seniors. Losing weight reduces pressure on the spine, making low-impact exercises more feasible and practical. These exercises, in turn, strengthen muscles that support proper posture, which helps prevent further strain on the spine and nerves.

When combined, these strategies offer seniors a well-rounded approach to sciatica relief. It's, however, essential to remember that progress may be gradual, and consistency is vital. By embracing these practices, seniors can experience reduced sciatic pain, improved spinal health, and a better quality of life as they navigate their golden years.

CHAPTER 4

NURTURING FLEXIBILITY AND MOBILITY FOR SENIORS

Maintaining flexibility and mobility becomes crucial for overall well-being as we age, especially among seniors. Gentle stretches and exercises tailored for seniors offer relief from aches and pains and enhance quality of life. These activities help maintain joint health, improve circulation, and contribute to better posture.

This chapter will delve into safe stretches and exercises and provide step-by-step instructions to ensure a comfortable and effective routine.

Flexibility — the range of motion around a joint, and mobility - the ability to move freely play pivotal roles in seniors' daily lives. They prevent stiffness, increase blood flow to muscles, and reduce the risk of injuries.

Also, maintaining flexibility and mobility can alleviate chronic pain caused by sciatica, Arthritis, and muscle imbalances.

For seniors, these benefits translate into an improved ability to perform daily activities, enhanced balance, and a reduced risk of falls. Flexibility and mobility also support independence, enabling seniors to enjoy their hobbies, stay active, and engage with their community.

Step-by-Step Instructions for Safe Stretches and Exercises for Seniors

- Find a comfortable and quiet space to perform your stretches and exercises. Wear loose, comfortable clothing that allows for easy movement.

- Start with a gentle warm-up, such as walking on the spot or gently moving your arms.

- Breathe deeply and evenly throughout the routine.

- Perform each stretch or exercise slowly and smoothly, without any jerking motions.

- Pay attention to your body's feedback; stretches should feel gentle and comfortable, not painful.

- Stop immediately and consult a healthcare professional if you experience pain or discomfort.

As you progress, you can gradually increase the duration

or repetitions.

Knee to Chest

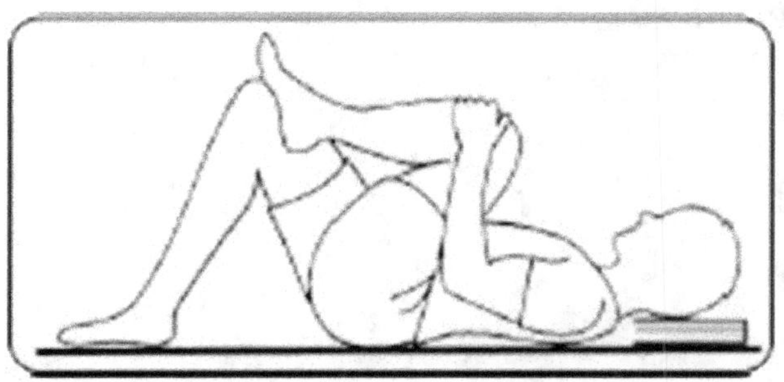

Knee to Chest Exercise

- Lie down with your knees bent and feet flat on the floor, approximately hip-width apart. Raise your head slightly using a book or flat cushion

- Relax your shoulders and tuck your chin in

- Slowly pull one knee up toward your chest

- Hold for 20–30 seconds before slowly returning your foot to the floor and repeat with the opposite leg

- Repeat 2–3 times on each side

Sciatic Mobilizer

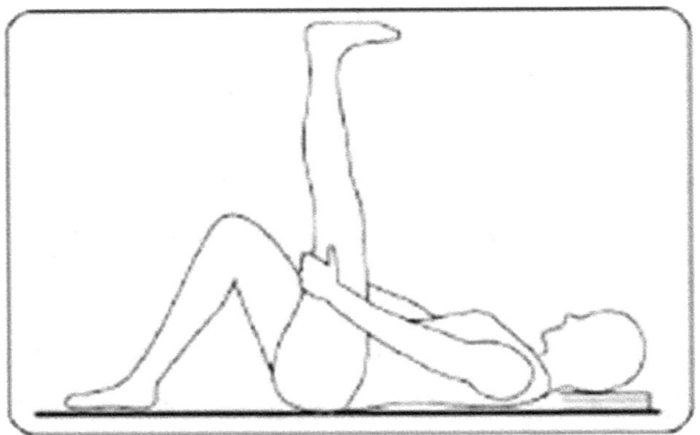

Sciatic Mobilizer

- Lay down with your knees bent and feet flat, around hip-width apart

- Raise your head using a book or flat cushion

- Relax your shoulders and tuck your chin in

- Slowly pull one knee up toward your chest

- Hold onto the back of your thigh and slowly straighten your leg. Hold for 20–30 seconds

- Slowly return your foot to its original position and repeat with the opposite leg

- Hold for 20–30 seconds

- Slowly release and repeat with the opposite leg

- Repeat 2–3 times on each side

Gluteal Stretch

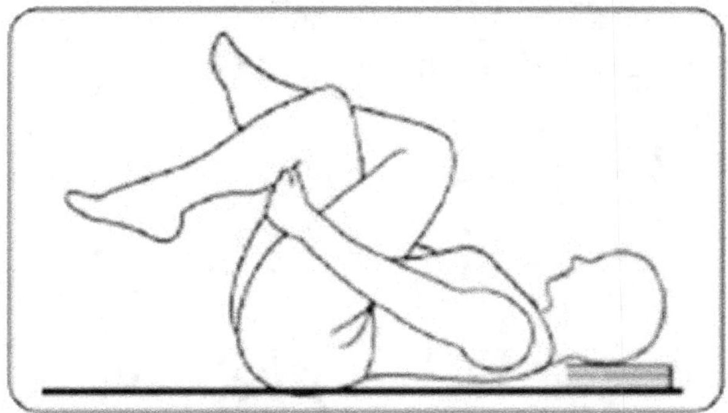

Gluteal Stretch

This deep stretch can be felt in the backs of the thighs and gluteal muscles (buttocks). These two areas are frequently affected by sciatica pain.

- Lie on the floor with your knees bent, feet flat, and hip-width apart

- Raise your head using a book, yoga block, or flat cushion

- Relax your shoulders and tuck in your chin

- Slowly pull your left knee up and rest your ankle on your right thigh

- Loop your hands around your right thigh and pull the leg up toward your chest.

- Keep your lower back on the floor and your hips straight.

- Hold for up to 20-30 seconds. Slowly release and repeat with the opposite leg

- Repeat 2-3 times on each side

Back Extension

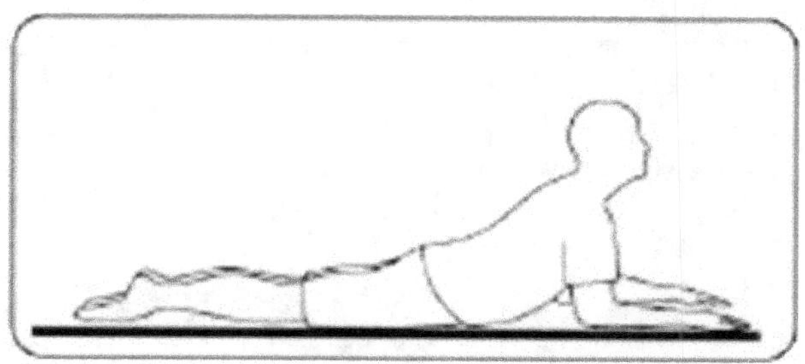

Back Extension

This is an excellent stretch for lower back pain and may be especially helpful if a prolapsed disc causes your symptoms.

- Lie on your stomach with your forearms on the floor, elbows bent and tucked into your sides

- Keep your neck straight and your lower body relaxed

- Keeping your forearms on the floor, slowly push up and arch your back gently.

- Hold for 20–30 seconds. Repeat 8–10 times

Hamstring Stretch

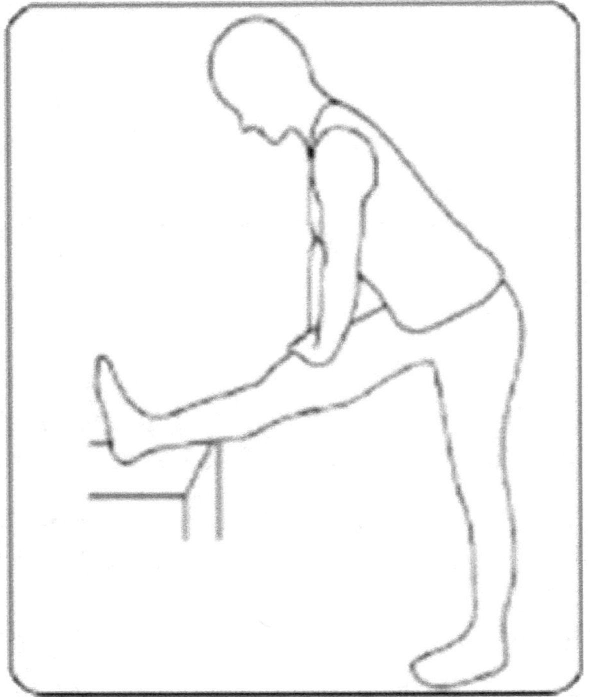

Hamstring Stretch

- In a standing position, raise one foot on a solid surface, such as a step

- Point your toes upward and keep your leg straight, slowly lean forward, keeping your back straight

- Hold for 5–10 seconds, then relax

- Return your foot to the floor and repeat with the

opposite leg

- Repeat 2–3 times on each side

When to do Your Sciatica Exercises

Doing these stretches several times daily for the best results would be best. Although it can be time-consuming, this is the best way to ensure that your sciatica exercises are practical and worthwhile.

Gentle stretches and exercises tailored for seniors are essential for maintaining flexibility and mobility, which are fundamental for a healthy and active lifestyle. These activities can alleviate discomfort, improve posture, and enhance overall well-being.

By incorporating safe stretches and exercises into your daily routine and following step-by-step instructions, you'll take proactive steps toward nurturing your body's flexibility, mobility, and vitality as you embrace your senior years.

Always consult a healthcare professional before beginning any new exercise regimen, especially if you have existing health conditions.

CHAPTER 5

A HOLISTIC APPROACH TO PAIN MANAGEMENT

Sciatic pain is often characterized by discomfort radiating along the sciatic nerve, which can be a debilitating experience.

While seeking medical advice is paramount, there are effective techniques you can incorporate into your daily routine to alleviate the pain and improve your quality of life.

This chapter will explore three holistic approaches: utilizing heat and cold therapy, practicing breathing exercises and relaxation techniques, and embracing mindfulness and meditation.

Heat and Cold Therapy

Heat and cold therapy can relieve sciatic pain by altering blood flow, reducing inflammation, and relaxing muscles. Applying heat, such as a warm compress or heating pad, can help increase circulation to the affected area and ease tense muscles. Conversely, cold therapy can numb the area, reduce swelling, and alleviate pain.

Remember: Place a barrier between the source and your skin to prevent burns or frostbite.

Breathing Exercises and Relaxation Techniques
Deep breathing and relaxation exercises play a crucial role
in pain management. They help your body release tension,
reduce stress, and improve oxygen flow, which can aid in the
healing process. Practicing deep, slow breaths can activate
the body's relaxation response, calming both the mind
and the muscles affected by sciatic pain. Techniques like
diaphragmatic breathing or progressive muscle relaxation
can be practical tools in your pain management arsenal.

How to incorporate this technique:

- Find a quiet and comfortable space to sit or lie down.

- Close your eyes and take slow, deep breaths through
  your nose and mouth.

- Focus on the rise and fall of your abdomen as you
  breathe deeply.

- As you exhale, release any tension or stress from your
  body.

Mindfulness and Meditation Practices
Mindfulness and meditation offer powerful tools for
controlling pain perception and promoting overall
well-being. You can redirect your attention away from the
pain by training your mind to focus on the present moment.

Mindfulness teaches you to acknowledge the discomfort
without judgment, which can reduce the anxiety that often
accompanies chronic pain. Conversely, meditation helps

cultivate a sense of calm and inner peace, making it easier to cope with sciatic pain.

How to incorporate this technique.

- Sit or lie down in a comfortable position.

- Focus on your breath or a specific sensation in your body.

- When your mind wanders, gently bring your focus back to your chosen engagement point.

Start with a few minutes and gradually increase the duration as you become more comfortable. Effectively managing sciatic pain requires a multifaceted approach that addresses not only the physical discomfort but also the emotional and mental aspects.

Utilizing heat and cold therapy, practicing breathing exercises and relaxation techniques, and embracing mindfulness and meditation can empower you to take control of your pain and enhance your well-being.

Remember that everyone's experience with sciatic pain is unique, so finding the best combination of techniques for you is essential.

Always consult a healthcare professional before starting any new pain management regimen. With dedication and patience, you can discover relief and regain a sense of comfort and tranquillity amidst the challenges of sciatic pain.

BEFORE WE CONTINUE...

I hope you're enjoying the journey so far!

If this book has resonated with you in any way, I'd be incredibly grateful if you could take a moment to leave an honest review on Amazon. You can leave a review by either scanning this QR code or following the link below; then scroll down to
Review This Product

https://geni.us/B0CG3RT393

Now, let's get back to it...

CHAPTER 6

HERBAL AND SUPPLEMENT REMEDIES

For those seeking alternative methods to manage sciatic pain, herbal remedies, and supplements offer a natural approach that has gained attention for its potential effectiveness.

Herbs such as Turmeric, Ginger, and Devil's Claw have long been used in traditional medicine for their anti-inflammatory and pain-relieving properties.

However, it's essential to navigate this path with awareness and caution.

In this chapter, we'll delve into herbal remedies and supplements for sciatic pain, discussing their benefits, precautions, and the significance of consulting a healthcare professional before introducing any new accessories to your regimen.

Natural Remedies

- Turmeric contains an active compound called curcumin, which has potent anti-inflammatory properties. It can help reduce inflammation that may contribute to sciatic pain. Curcumin's potential pain-relieving effects are similar to non-steroidal

anti-inflammatory drugs (NSAIDs) but without the
possible side effects. Turmeric can be consumed as
a spice in food or taken as a supplement.

- Ginger is known for its anti-inflammatory and
  analgesic properties. It may help alleviate pain
  associated with sciatica by reducing inflammation
  and improving circulation. Ginger can be consumed
  in various forms, including fresh ginger root, tea, or
  supplements.

- Devil's Claw is a plant native to Africa and has been
  used for centuries to manage pain and inflammation.
  Its active compounds, called iridoid glycosides, are
  believed to have anti-inflammatory effects.

While herbal remedies offer potential benefits for sciatic
pain relief, it's essential to approach them with caution
and awareness of potential risks. Regular check-ins
with a healthcare provider allow you to discuss your
experience with herbal supplements and make any
necessary adjustments to your treatment plan.

Benefits of Herbal Supplements

- Natural Approach - Herbal remedies provide an
  alternative to conventional medications, appealing to
  those who prefer a more natural approach to pain
  management.

- Anti-Inflammatory Properties - Many herbs used
  for sciatic pain relief possess anti-inflammatory
  properties, which can help reduce inflammation that
  contributes to pain.

- Minimal Side Effects - When used correctly, herbal supplements often have fewer side effects than pharmaceutical ones.

Precautions for Herbal Supplements

- Interaction with Medications: Herbal supplements can interact with prescription medications, potentially affecting their efficacy or causing adverse effects.

- Allergic Reactions: Allergies to herbs are possible, so it's crucial to be aware of any potential allergic reactions when introducing a new supplement.

- Dosage and Quality: Herbal supplements vary in quality and potency. Proper dosage and using high-quality products are essential for achieving desired results.

Before introducing any herbal supplement into your sciatic pain management routine, consulting a healthcare professional is essential.

Here's why:

- Personalized Guidance: A healthcare provider can help determine whether herbal supplements are appropriate for your health, considering any existing medical conditions, medications, or allergies.

- Avoiding Interactions: Healthcare professionals can evaluate potential interactions between herbal supplements and any prescription medications you may take, ensuring your safety.

- Proper Dosage: Professionals can guide the appropriate dosage of herbal supplements to ensure their effectiveness and minimize potential side effects.

By combining traditional remedies' wisdom with modern health care expertise, you can confidently navigate the path of herbal supplements, empowering yourself to find effective and natural relief from sciatic pain.

However, caution is paramount. Always consult a healthcare professional before introducing any new supplements, as they can provide personalized guidance, assess potential interactions, and ensure your safety.

In conclusion, herbal remedies and supplements offer a natural and appealing option for managing sciatic pain.

With herbs like Turmeric, Ginger, and Devil's Claw showcasing potential anti-inflammatory and pain-relieving properties, it's no wonder many individuals turn to these alternatives.

CHAPTER 7

NATURE'S SOOTHING TONIC FOR RELIEF

In today's fast-paced world, finding holistic approaches to health and wellness has gained immense popularity.

Aromatherapy is an age-old practice that utilizes essential oils for their therapeutic benefits. It has emerged as a powerful tool for promoting relaxation, alleviating pain, and enhancing overall well-being. With a history dating back to ancient civilizations, aromatherapy continues to captivate individuals seeking natural alternatives to conventional treatments.

This chapter will delve into aromatherapy and essential oils, focusing on their role in pain relief and their complementary potential alongside other treatments and safe usage methods for seniors.

The Fragrant Path to Comfort and Pain Relief.
Nature has gifted us a treasure trove of aromatic plants with remarkable healing properties.

Essential oils, extracted through methods like steam distillation and cold pressing, capture the concentrated essence of these plants. When used correctly, these oils can offer profound relief from various types of pain.

Peppermint oil is a versatile essential oil often used for pain relief. Its cooling sensation can provide immediate relief from tension headaches and is beneficial for soothing sore muscles and joints.

With its potent anti-inflammatory properties,

Eucalyptus oil can be particularly effective for respiratory discomfort, making it a go-to choice for those suffering from congestion or sinus-related pain.

Aromatherapy as a complement to other treatments.
Aromatherapy isn't just about the pleasant scents; it has a deep-rooted connection with our emotional and mental well-being. Aromatherapy can enhance effectiveness and contribute to a holistic healing experience when incorporated alongside other therapies. For example, cancer patients undergoing chemotherapy often experience nausea and discomfort.

Studies have shown that inhaling ginger or lemon essential oil can help alleviate these side effects and improve their overall quality of life.

Furthermore, aromatherapy can be pivotal in managing chronic pain conditions like Arthritis. When used with traditional pain management strategies, such as medications or physical therapy, essential oils like frankincense, chamomile, and marjoram can provide additional relief.

The relaxing aroma of these oils can help reduce stress and anxiety and is known to exacerbate chronic pain. This highlights the potential of aromatherapy as a supportive and complementary tool in the broader healthcare landscape.

Safe Methods of Using Essential Oils for Seniors
As our bodies age, they become more sensitive, and specific precautions need to be taken when using essential oils, especially for seniors.

Some essential oils might be more suitable for seniors due to their gentle nature. Oils like lavender, chamomile, and bergamot are generally considered safe options.

Here are some safe methods for incorporating aromatherapy into the lives of older adults:

- Dilution - Essential oils are highly concentrated and can cause skin irritation if applied directly. For seniors, it's crucial to dilute essential oils in a carrier oil like coconut or jojoba oil before applying them to the skin. A general guideline is to use 1-2 drops of essential oil per teaspoon of carrier oil.

- Inhalation - Diffusing essential oils is a safe way for seniors to experience their benefits. An ultrasonic diffuser, which releases a fine mist of oil and water into the air, helps maintain a controlled and gentle aroma in the room.

- Topical Application - When applying essential oils topically, choosing areas with good blood circulation, such as the wrists or the soles of the feet, is recommended. Always perform a patch test before using a new essential oil to avoid adverse reactions.

- Consultation - Before introducing aromatherapy into a senior's routine, it's wise to consult with a healthcare professional, especially if they have underlying medical conditions or are taking medications that could interact with the oils.

As with any holistic practice, it's essential to approach aromatherapy with care and mindfulness, particularly when considering its application for seniors.

In conclusion, aromatherapy and essential oils offer a fragrant pathway to pain relief, relaxation, and overall wellness. With their rich history and extensive therapeutic benefits, these oils have firmly established themselves as valuable tools in holistic healing. Their potential to complement traditional treatments and their versatility in managing various types of pain makes them a popular choice for those seeking natural alternatives.

CHAPTER 8

ACUPUNCTURE, ACUPRESSURE, CHIROPRACTIC REMEDIES

Acupressure, non-invasive and gentle, can also help reduce pain and promote relaxation, making it seniors who may be wary of needles.

As we age, prioritizing our physical and mental well-being becomes increasingly essential. While conventional medical treatments are crucial in senior healthcare, many individuals are exploring holistic approaches to complement traditional methods.

Acupuncture, acupressure, chiropractic care, and massage therapy are four such practices that offer seniors natural and effective ways to manage pain, enhance mobility, and improve overall quality of life.

Additionally, these practices can address issues commonly associated with aging, such as sleep disturbances and digestive problems. Acupuncture improves sleep quality by regulating the body's internal clock. Acupressure can help alleviate indigestion and constipation by stimulating digestive points.

Acupuncture and Acupressure

Acupuncture and acupressure, ancient wisdom for modern aging, is rooted in ancient Chinese medicine, based on the concept of energy flow, or "qi," through pathways known as meridians.

These practices aim to restore balance in the body by stimulating specific points along these meridians. While acupuncture involves inserting thin needles into these points, acupressure applies pressure to the same issues using fingers, thumbs, or devices.

For seniors, acupuncture and acupressure can offer a multitude of benefits. One of the most significant advantages is pain relief. Many older adults experience chronic pain due to Arthritis, joint stiffness, and muscle tension.

Acupuncture is known to release endorphins, the body's natural painkillers, relieving various types of pain.

Chiropractic Care and Spinal Adjustments

Aligning seniors with comfort through chiropractic care primarily focuses on diagnosing and treating musculoskeletal disorders through spinal adjustments.

As we age, our spine undergoes changes that can lead to misalignments, nerve compression, and reduced mobility. Chiropractors specialize in realigning the spine and improving joint function, which can alleviate pain and enhance the physical process.

For seniors with chronic back pain, spinal adjustments offer a non-invasive alternative to surgery or medication.

Chiropractors use controlled, gentle force to correct misalignments, allowing the body's natural healing processes to take over. These adjustments can lead to improved mobility, reduced pain, and a better quality of life for older adults.

Moreover, chiropractic care is not only about spinal adjustments. It often encompasses lifestyle guidance, exercises, and nutritional advice tailored to seniors' needs. This comprehensive approach can improve overall health, mobility, and independence.

Massage therapy is a well-known practice for relaxation and stress reduction. However, its benefits extend far beyond that, especially for seniors. As we age, our bodies experience decreased circulation, muscle stiffness, and joint pain. Massage therapy addresses these concerns by promoting blood flow, releasing muscle tension, and improving flexibility.

Safety Considerations for Seniors
While these holistic practices offer numerous benefits, seniors need to approach them with caution and under professional guidance:

- Consultation - Before undergoing any of these therapies, seniors should consult with their healthcare provider, especially if they have pre-existing medical conditions or are taking medications.

- Qualified Practitioners - Seek out licensed and experienced practitioners in acupuncture, chiropractic care, and massage therapy with specific expertise in working with seniors.

- Communication - Communicate your health history,

concerns, and comfort level with the practitioner to ensure the treatment is tailored to your needs.

- Dosage - Seniors might require treatment duration and intensity adjustments. Start with shorter sessions and gradually increase as your body adjusts.

- Feedback - Throughout the treatment, provide feedback to the practitioner regarding your comfort level and any sensations you experience.

Acupuncture, acupressure, chiropractic care, and massage therapy offer various benefits, from pain relief to enhanced mobility and emotional well-being. Deeply rooted in ancient traditions, these practices provide seniors practical tools to support their overall health.

However, seniors must prioritize safety by consulting healthcare professionals and choosing qualified practitioners to ensure a positive and beneficial experience.

In conclusion, as the population ages, holistic approaches to senior wellness are gaining recognition for their potential to improve physical and mental well-being.

CHAPTER 9

YOGA, TAI CHI, AND THE ART OF INTEGRATION

By embracing these holistic methods, seniors can embark on a journey of improved vitality, comfort, and quality of life in their golden years.

Our bodies undergo various changes with age, leading to discomfort and reduced mobility. Seniors, in particular, often face challenges such as sciatica, balance issues, and chronic pain.

Fortunately, yoga and tai chi offer tailored solutions to address these concerns and promote overall well-being. Integrating these ancient arts into daily routines can bring about profound improvements in physical health, balance, and pain relief for seniors.

Yoga Poses for Seniors with Sciatica
Sciatica, characterized by pain radiating along the sciatic nerve, can significantly impact seniors' quality of life. Yoga emphasizes gentle stretches, controlled breathing, and mindful movement, which can relieve sciatic pain and improve flexibility.

Certain yoga poses can be particularly beneficial for seniors with sciatica.

The Child's Pose (Balasana) is a gentle stretch that can provide relief by lengthening the spine and relieving pressure on the sciatic nerve.

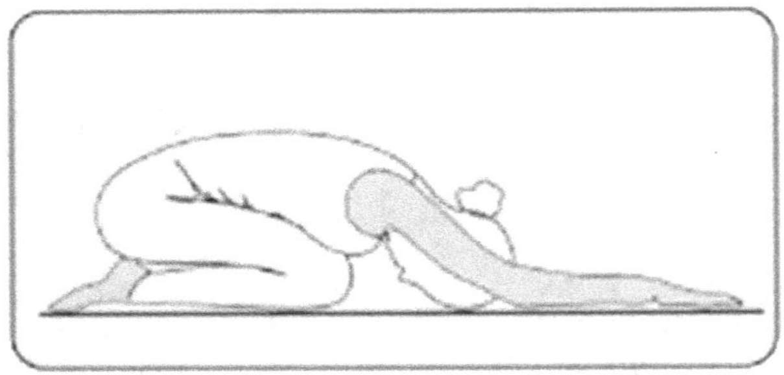

The Child's or Balasana Pose

- Place your hands and knees on the yoga mat.

- Spread your knees as wide as your mat, keeping the tops of your feet on the floor with the big toes touching.

- Rest your belly between your thighs and place your forehead on the floor.

- Relax the shoulders, jaw, and eyes. If placing the forehead on the floor is uncomfortable, rest it on a block or two stacked fists. An energy point at the centre of the forehead in between the eyebrows stimulates the vagus nerve. It supports a "rest and digest" response. Finding a comfortable place for the forehead is critical to gaining this soothing benefit.

- Stretch your arms in front of you with the palms toward the floor, or bring your arms back alongside your thighs with the palms facing upwards. You can also stretch the arms forward with palms facing up for a shoulder release or try bending the elbows so that the palms touch and rest the thumbs at the back of the neck. In this position, move the elbows forward. Stay as long as you like, eventually reconnecting with your breath's steady inhales and exhales.

The benefit of Child's Pose is a gentle stretch for the shoulders, back, hips, thighs, neck, and ankles, and it can help relieve sciatic pain and promote deep breathing, mindfulness, and relaxation.

Evidence has shown that slow breathing can lower blood pressure and improve lung function and respiratory fitness.

Learning to use this pose wisely is the part of your developing practice where you listen to your body's inner voice and do what it tells you. Your body will notify you when to rest.

It might need different things on different days.

Keeping your ear finely tuned to the messages your body sends you and respectfully responding to them is the most incredible lesson the child's pose offers. You will come to know when to use Child's Pose during your yoga practice.

The Cat-Cow Stretch helps warm up the spine and increases spinal flexibility.

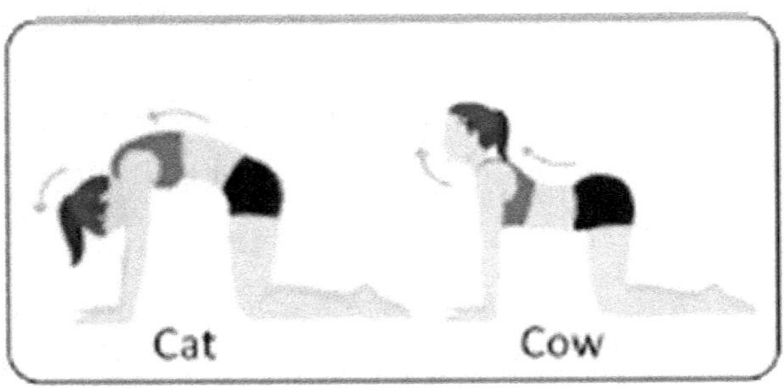

Cat-Cow Stretch

- Start on your hands and knees, aligning your wrists underneath your shoulders and your knees underneath your hips.

- Think of the spine as a straight line connecting the shoulders to the hips. Try visualizing the line extending forward through the crown of the head and back through the tailbone. This is the position of a neutral spine. It is keeping the neck long by looking down and out.

Inhale and Arch for Cow Pose

- Tilt your pelvis back so that your tailbone sticks up. Let this movement ripple from your tailbone up your spine so that your neck is the last thing to move.

- Your belly drops, but keep your abdominal muscles hugging your spine by drawing your navel in.

- Take your gaze gently up toward the ceiling without cranking your neck.

Exhale and Round for Cat Pose

- Release the tops of your feet to the floor.

- Tip your pelvis forward, tucking your tailbone. Again, let this action move up your spine, which will naturally round.

- Draw your navel toward your spine.

- Drop your head.

- Take your gaze to your navel.

Repeat the Cat-Cow Stretch on each inhale and exhale, matching the movement with your breathing.

The Cobra Pose
The benefit of the Cobra Pose is that it increases the spine's mobility, strengthens spinal support muscles, and can help relieve back pain. It opens the chest and the front of the body. This can be particularly helpful if you sit for much of the day. Sitting leads to tight chest muscles and stretched, weakened back muscles. Cobra can counteract that hunched-over posture.

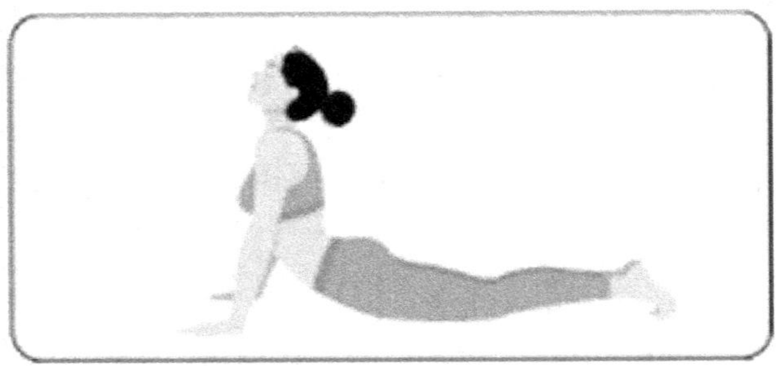

Cobra or Bhujangasana Pose

- Begin by laying down flat on your stomach.

- Place your palms flat on the ground directly under your shoulders. Bend your elbows straight back and hug them into your sides.

- Pause momentarily, looking straight down at your mat with your neck in a neutral position. Anchor your pubic bone to the floor.

- Inhale to lift your chest off the floor. Roll your shoulders back and keep your low ribs on the floor.

- Make sure your elbows continue hugging your sides. Don't let them wing out to either side.

- Keep your neck neutral. Don't crank it up. Your gaze should stay on the floor.

- Exhale to release back to the floor.

Tai Chi – Balancing Act for Seniors.
Tai chi, an ancient Chinese martial art characterized by slow and flowing movements, is particularly suitable for older adults with balance issues or fear of falling.

The benefits of Tai Chi Balance for seniors include

- Balance Improvement - The deliberate, controlled Tai Chi movements help seniors develop a stronger sense of balance and stability. They can significantly reduce the risk of falls, which can be especially dangerous for older individuals.

- Pain Relief - The fluid movements of tai chi can enhance joint flexibility and muscle strength, potentially relieving chronic pain conditions like arthritis.

- Mind-Body Connection - Tai chi encourages mindfulness and concentration, fostering a solid mind-body connection, and can contribute to reduced stress and improved mental well-being.

Integrating Yoga and Tai Chi into Daily Routines
The true magic of yoga and tai chi lies in their integration into daily routines.

Seniors can seamlessly incorporate these practices for maximum benefits

- Morning Wake-Up Routine - Begin the day with gentle stretches and tai chi movements. Focus on deep breathing and gentle movement to wake up the body and calm the mind.

- Midday Energizer - Taking short breaks during the day to perform a few simple yoga poses or tai chi movements can help alleviate stiffness, improve circulation, and boost energy levels.

- Evening Relaxation - Wind down in the evening with a restorative yoga or tai chi practice.

- Consistency - The benefits of yoga and tai chi come with consistent practice. Aim for regular exercise to experience meaningful improvements in your well-being.

- Emphasize relaxation and deep breathing to prepare for a peaceful night's sleep.

- Breathing Exercises - Incorporate deep breathing exercises from both practices whenever needed. Deep, mindful breathing can help manage stress, improve oxygenation, and promote relaxation.

- Social Engagement - Consider joining a local yoga or tai chi class tailored for seniors. Engaging in group activities not only offers physical benefits but also provides a sense of community and companionship.

- Professional Guidance - When starting any new exercise regimen, it's advisable to consult a healthcare provider, especially if you have underlying health conditions.

- Qualified Instructors - Seek certified instructors with experience working with seniors. They can offer personalized modifications and ensure proper alignment to prevent injury.

- Modifications - Always listen to your body and make modifications as needed. It's important to practice within your comfort zone and avoid pushing yourself too hard.

- Progression - Gradually increase the intensity and

duration of your practice as your body becomes more accustomed to the movements.

These practices offer tailored solutions to address common concerns such as sciatica, balance issues, and chronic pain. Their gentle movements focus on breath and emphasize mindfulness.

Yoga and tai chi provide holistic benefits beyond the physical realm. By approaching these practices with an open mind, seeking professional guidance, and integrating them into daily routines, seniors can embark on improved physical health, enhanced balance, and a greater sense of overall well-being in their golden years.

In conclusion, integrating yoga and tai chi into daily routines can bring about transformative changes in the lives of seniors.

CHAPTER 10

A GUIDE TO ERGONOMIC AIDS

As individuals age, maintaining comfort, mobility, and independence becomes paramount. Thankfully, advancements in ergonomic aids and assistive tools have paved the way for seniors to enjoy a higher quality of life.

From ergonomic cushions and chairs that promote improved posture to walking aids that reduce strain and assistive tools for daily activities, many options exist to enhance well-being and ensure seniors can continue to engage actively in their daily lives.

Benefits of Ergonomic Cushions and Chairs:

- Spinal Alignment - Ergonomic cushions and chairs are designed to align the spine correctly, reducing the strain on back muscles and promoting a neutral posture.

- Pressure Relief - Memory foam cushions and gel-infused seats distribute weight evenly, reducing pressure points and the risk of developing pressure ulcers.

- Improved Circulation - Ergonomic cushions can help improve blood circulation by preventing compression of blood vessels and reducing the risk of swelling.

- Customizable Support - Many ergonomic chairs and cushions come with adjustable features, allowing users to tailor the support to their needs.

- Walking Aids and Devices - Enhancing mobility and reducing strain

For seniors, maintaining mobility is vital to enjoying an active lifestyle. Walking aids and devices are essential tools that provide support, stability, and confidence for those with mobility challenges.

Types of Walking Aids:

- Canes - Canes provide additional support while walking and helping distribute weight evenly. They come in various styles, including single-point and quad-point walking canes for added stability.

- Walkers - Walkers offer more comprehensive support and stability, making them ideal for seniors who require additional balance assistance.

- Spinal Alignment - Ergonomic cushions and chairs are designed to align the spine correctly, reducing the strain on back muscles and promoting a neutral posture.

- Rollators - Rollators combine the benefits of walkers with wheels, allowing users to move more freely while maintaining stability.

- Crutches -Crutches are often used for individuals

recovering from injuries or surgeries. They provide
support by transferring weight from the legs to the
upper body.

- Reacher Grabbers - Reacher grabbers help seniors
pick up objects from the ground or shelves without
bending over or straining.

- Adaptive Eating Utensils - These are designed with
ergonomic handles and features that make eating
easier for individuals with limited dexterity.

- Jar and Bottle Openers - These tools provide extra
grip and leverage, making opening tight lids on jars
and bottles easier.

- Button Hooks and Zipper Pulls - These tools assist
with fastening buttons and zippers, allowing seniors
to dress more independently.

- Adaptive Gardening Tools - Seniors who enjoy
gardening can benefit from ergonomic gardening
tools designed to reduce strain on joints and muscles.

Integration and Implementation.
Choosing the right ergonomic aids and assistive tools is vital,
but integrating them effectively into daily routines is equally
essential.

Here's how to ensure seniors make the most of these
supportive devices we would suggest:

- Professional Consultation - Before investing in
ergonomic aids, consider consulting a healthcare
professional or occupational therapist. They can

guide the most suitable options based on individual needs.

- Proper Fitting - Ensure that walking aids are adjusted to the correct height and offer a comfortable grip. Ill-fitting devices can lead to discomfort and potential injuries.

- Training and Practice - Seniors should receive proper training on using walking aids.

- Regular Maintenance: Keep ergonomic chairs, cushions, and walking aids in good condition through regular maintenance and adjustments.

- Gradual Transition: Transitioning gradually is vital for individuals new to using assistive tools. Start by using them in familiar environments before venturing out.

- Regular Evaluation: As seniors' needs change, it's important to regularly evaluate the effectiveness of ergonomic aids and assistive tools and adjust accordingly.

Promoting Well-Being and Independence
Ergonomic aids and assistive tools enhance seniors' comfort, mobility, and independence. These tools are not only practical but also empower individuals to engage actively in their daily lives and maintain their sense of dignity.

By choosing the correct aids, seeking professional guidance, and integrating them seamlessly into daily routines, seniors can enjoy a higher quality of life, reduced strain, and the freedom to participate in activities they love. Ultimately, these tools are bridges to a more comfortable and fulfilling journey through the golden years.

Chapter 11

Conclusion

In this final chapter of our journey through the pages of this book, we conclude—an endpoint that is, but also, in many ways, a new beginning with the information we have gained. Throughout these chapters, we've delved into the world of sciatica, exploring its causes, symptoms, and the intricate ways it can impact the lives of seniors.

While consulting a healthcare professional is crucial for accurate diagnosis and guidance, incorporating natural treatments into your routine can complement traditional approaches.

Here's a comprehensive plan to manage sciatica while maintaining consistency and adapting strategies as you age.

Yoga for Flexibility
Participate in gentle yoga classes tailored for seniors. Yoga can help improve flexibility, strengthen core muscles, and alleviate sciatic pain. Choose poses that open the hips and stretch the hamstrings, such as the Child's Pose, Cat-Cow Stretch, and Supine Hand-to-Big-Toe Pose.

Warm Compresses and Cold Packs
Apply warm compresses or heating pads to the affected area to relax muscles and promote blood flow. Alternatively,

use cold packs to reduce inflammation and numb the area temporarily.

Mind-Body Techniques
Practice mindfulness meditation and deep breathing exercises to manage stress, which can exacerbate sciatic pain. Mind-body techniques can help you stay mentally resilient and cope with the challenges of managing chronic pain.

Ergonomic Support
Invest in ergonomic cushions and chairs that support proper posture and alleviate pressure on the sciatic nerve. As you age, periodically assess the need for additional ergonomic support to accommodate any changes in mobility.

Hydrotherapy and Massage
Consider hydrotherapy, such as warm baths or pool exercises, to relax muscles and reduce pain. Regular massages can help relieve tension and improve blood circulation. Opt for gentle techniques that cater to your age and comfort level.

Age-Adaptive Modifications
Some exercises or stretches become challenging as you age. Work with a physical therapist to modify your routine and adapt to your changing needs. Regularly reassess your treatment plan and adjust it based on your body's response and any age-related changes.

Lifestyle Adjustments
Maintain a healthy weight to reduce pressure on the spine and nerves. Avoid prolonged sitting or standing, and take regular breaks to move around and stretch.

Social Support and Mental Well-Being
Engage in social activities and hobbies that bring you joy.

Staying socially connected can positively impact your mental well-being. Seek support from friends, family, or support groups to share experiences and coping strategies.

Surgical Consideration
Discuss surgical options with your healthcare provider if natural treatments no longer provide relief and the condition worsens with age. Age-related considerations, risks, and benefits will guide the decision.

Acceptance and Adaptation Discs
Embrace that managing sciatica is a journey that might require ongoing adjustments as you age. Approach your treatment plan with patience, flexibility, and the understanding that your body's needs may change over time.

Remember that every individual's experience with sciatica is unique, and there is no one-size-fits-all approach.

Combining natural treatments with age-adaptive strategies and professional guidance allows you to manage sciatica effectively while maintaining your comfort and quality of life throughout aging.

You are not defined by your condition but by your spirit, resilience, and capacity to thrive. The journey continues, and you can shape it as you choose.

Regular Check-Ins with Healthcare Providers
Schedule regular check-ins with your healthcare provider to monitor your progress and adjust your treatment plan. Communicate any changes in symptoms, concerns, or challenges you might face as you age.

RESOURCE

The Natural Course of low back pain. Chiropractic Manual therapy, 2012 Vol20, page33

Exercise and Older Adults toolkit. (n.d.). National Institute on Aging. https://www.nia.nih.gov/exercisetoolkit

Ergonomics and Accommodations Pay Off | Arthritis Foundation. (n.d.).

https://www.arthritis.org/partnership/atwork/formanagers/ergonomics-and-accommodations

Turmeric. (n.d.). NCCIH.

https://www.nccih.nih.gov/health/turmeric

Ginger. (n.d.). NCCIH.

https://www.nccih.nih.gov/health/ginger

Devil's Claw: Overview, uses, side effects, precautions, interactions, dosing, and reviews. (n.d.).

https://www.webmd.com/vitamins/ai/ingredientmono984/devils-claw

Stress relief from laughter? It's no joke. (2021, July 29).

Mayo Clinic.
https://www.mayoclinic.org/healthylifestyle/stress-mana
gement/in-depth/stressrelief/art-20044456

Professional, C. C. M. (n.d.). Sciatica. Cleveland Clinic.

https://my.clevelandclinic.org/health/diseases/12792sciati
ca

Anti-Inflammatory diet Do's and Don'ts | Arthritis

Foundation. (n.d.).
https://www.arthritis.org/healthwellness/healthy-living/
nutrition/antiinflammatory/anti-inflammatory-diet

Better health. (n.d.).
https://aeawave.org/ArticlesMore/Better-Health/ArtMID
/1614/ArticleID/75

Hui, K. (2023). The five best shoes for Sciatica of 2023,

according to a podiatrist. LIVESTRONG.COM.

https://www.livestrong.com/article/13772577-bestshoes-f
or-sciatica/

A Quick Note from the Author

I hope you're enjoyed this book and found it helpful!
If this book has resonated with you in any way, I'd be
incredibly grateful if you could take a moment to leave an
honest review on Amazon.
Reviews don't just help other readers discover this book they
genuinely help me continue creating content I'm passionate
about. Even a sentence or two about what you've found
helpful makes a real difference.
You can leave a review by either scanning this QR code or
following the link below; then scroll down to **Review this
Product**

https://geni.us/B0CG3RT393

Thank you for being here and for your support.

**The LayPerson's Guides
Finally, guidebooks that speak your language.**

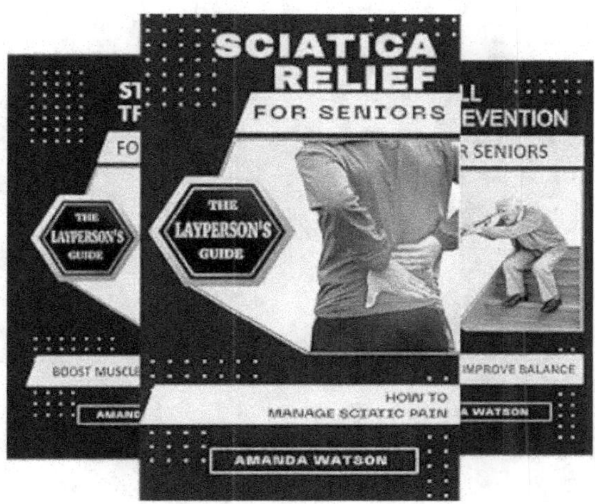

Also Available in Large Print

The Layperson Guides series is designed specifically for seniors who want clear, straightforward answers without the technical jargon or confusing terminology that fills most instruction manuals today. If you've ever felt overwhelmed by complicated directions, frustrated by assumptions that you already know the basics, or simply wished someone would explain things in plain English, this series is for you.

Each guide in this collection breaks down modern technology, everyday tasks, and practical skills into simple, easy-to-follow steps. There's no shame in wanting things explained clearly that's just good communication. These books respect your intelligence while recognizing that not everyone has grown up with smartphones, apps, and digital devices.

See More https://tinyurl.com/B0DR66HZS3

www.ingramcontent.com/pod-product-compliance
Lightning Source LLC
Chambersburg PA
CBHW070944250726

48663CB00001B/63